KMM's approach to mental health and wellness is unique and adaptive. Our goal is to provide insight into healthy eating habits, identifying foods that have the potential to trigger depression, anxiety, and foods that contribute to unhealthy emotions. The wellness side of our approach is to provide in-house activities, state-of-the-art journaling, workbooks, and seminars both corporate and one-on-one.

The authors, Reggie and Andrea are dedicated leaders in their communities with a heart to help people live healthier and peaceful lives. As a high-powered life coach and minister, Reggie understands the importance of clean eating, consistency, and the power of a changed mind. As an executive in her field of healthcare, a minister, and a high-powered life coach, Andrea's ultimate desire is to help people make quality decisions and provide hope to those who feel defeated by their circumstances.

Upon completion of the 21-day journal, you will have a better understanding of self-care, a healthier mindset, an appreciation for food alternatives and nutrition, and a strong resolve to address mental health and wellness. The daily affirmations, petitions, and acts of kindness will work wonders for you only if you are committed to making a change and believe in yourself. Affirmations are most effective when spoken aloud and or in front of a mirror. The recipes in this 21-day journal are intended to be a supplemental option only. Make no mistake, this journal is a powerful tool that will help you achieve your goals and transform your life from the inside out.

Disclaimer: The information provided in this book is for educational purposes only, and does not substitute for professional medical advice.

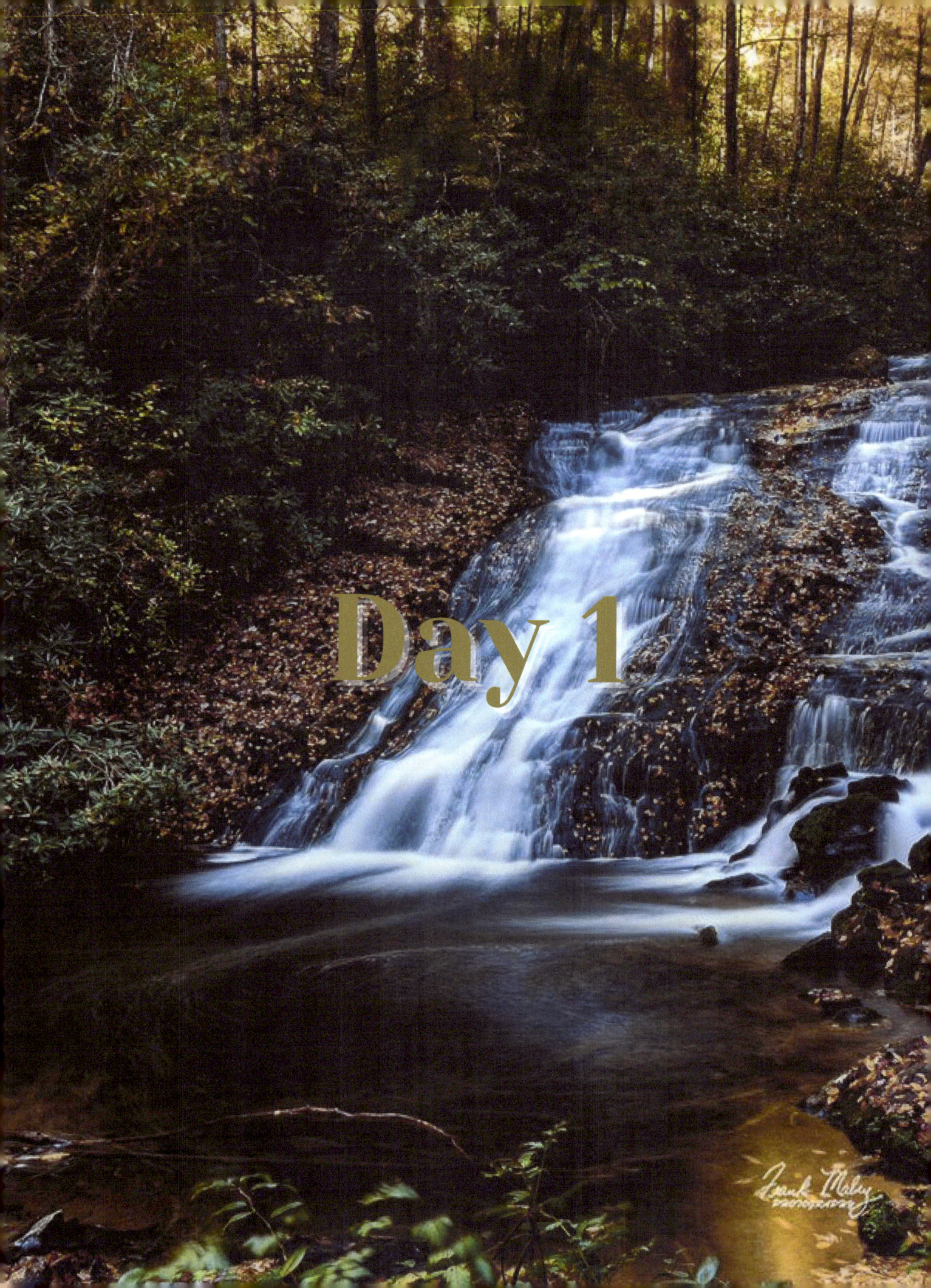

Daily affirmation:

Every day is new day full of hope, happiness and health.

Daily scripture:

"Anxiety in a man's heart weighs it down, but an encouraging word makes it glad." Proverbs 12:25

Daily Petition:

Father, I thank you for the positive changes in my life I am grateful for a fresh start in my life today.

Daily act of kindness:

Share with a person in need.

Nutritional recommendation:

Drink more water

Fact:

Asparagus is high in glutathione, an important anticarcinogen

Daily Journal

Day 2

Daily affirmation:

Only good things await me

Daily scripture:

Dear friend, I pray that you may enjoy health and that all may go well with you, even as your soul prospers. 3 John 1:2

Daily Petition:

'Keep and guard me as the pupil of your eye; hide me in the shadow of your wings.' Psalm 17:8

Daily act of kindness:

Give a compliment to 3 people

Nutritional recommendation:

Try a bowl of kimchi

Fact:

Broccoli contains selenium, a mineral that has been found to have anti-cancer and anti-viral properties

Daily Journal

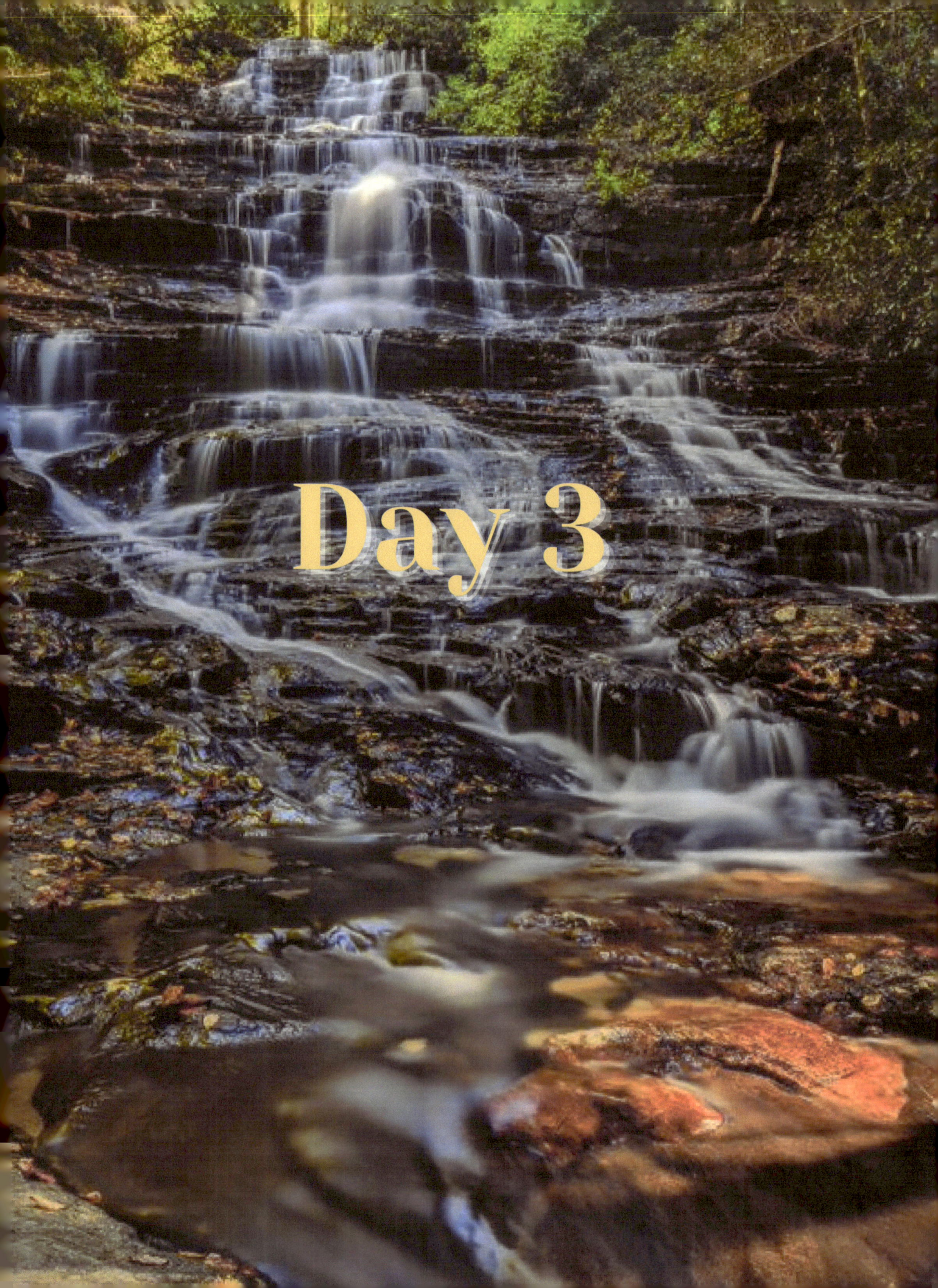

Daily affirmation:

I will take pride in my accomplishments today

Daily scripture:

"For I will restore health unto thee, and I will heal thee of thy wounds, saith the Lord, because thy called thee an Outcast," Jeremiah 30:17

Daily Petition:

You will show me the path of life; in your presence is fullness of joy, at your right hand there are pleasures forevermore. Psalm 16:11

Daily act of kindness:

Pay for someone's meal

Nutritional recommendation:

Eat more fresh fruit

FACT:

Chinese cabbage has anti-inflammatory properties

Daily Journal

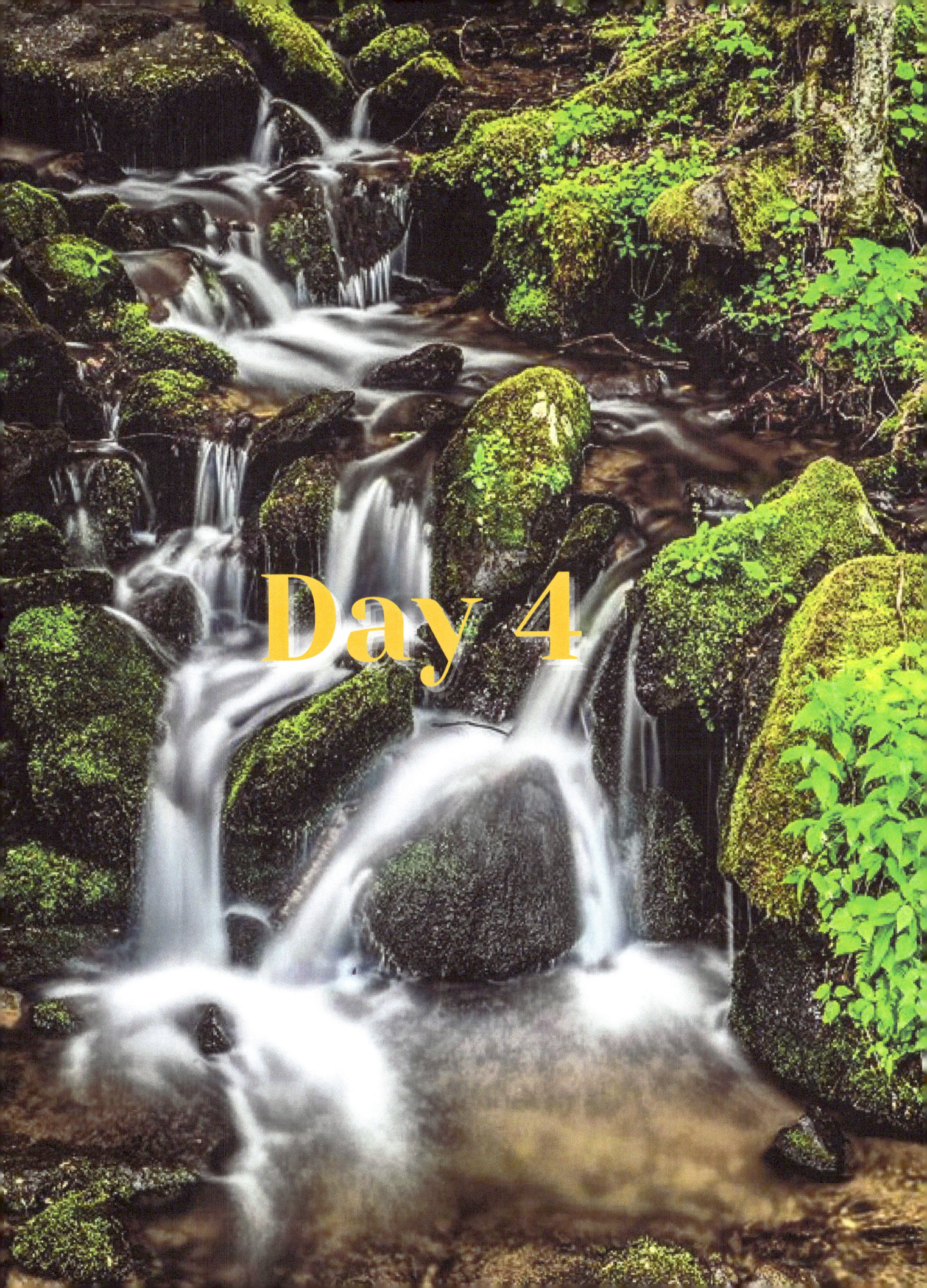

Daily affirmation:

I'm loved. I'm important. I'm unique.

Daily scripture:

"In God, I have put my trust; I will not be afraid. What can man do to me?" Psalms 56:11

Daily Petition:

Father, heal my heart and mind and restore your joy unto me.

Daily act of kindness:

Say something kind to a friend or stranger

Nutritional recommendation:

Try baked fish or chicken

FACT:

Kale contains lutein and zeaxanthin, which protect the eyes from macular degeneration

Daily Journal

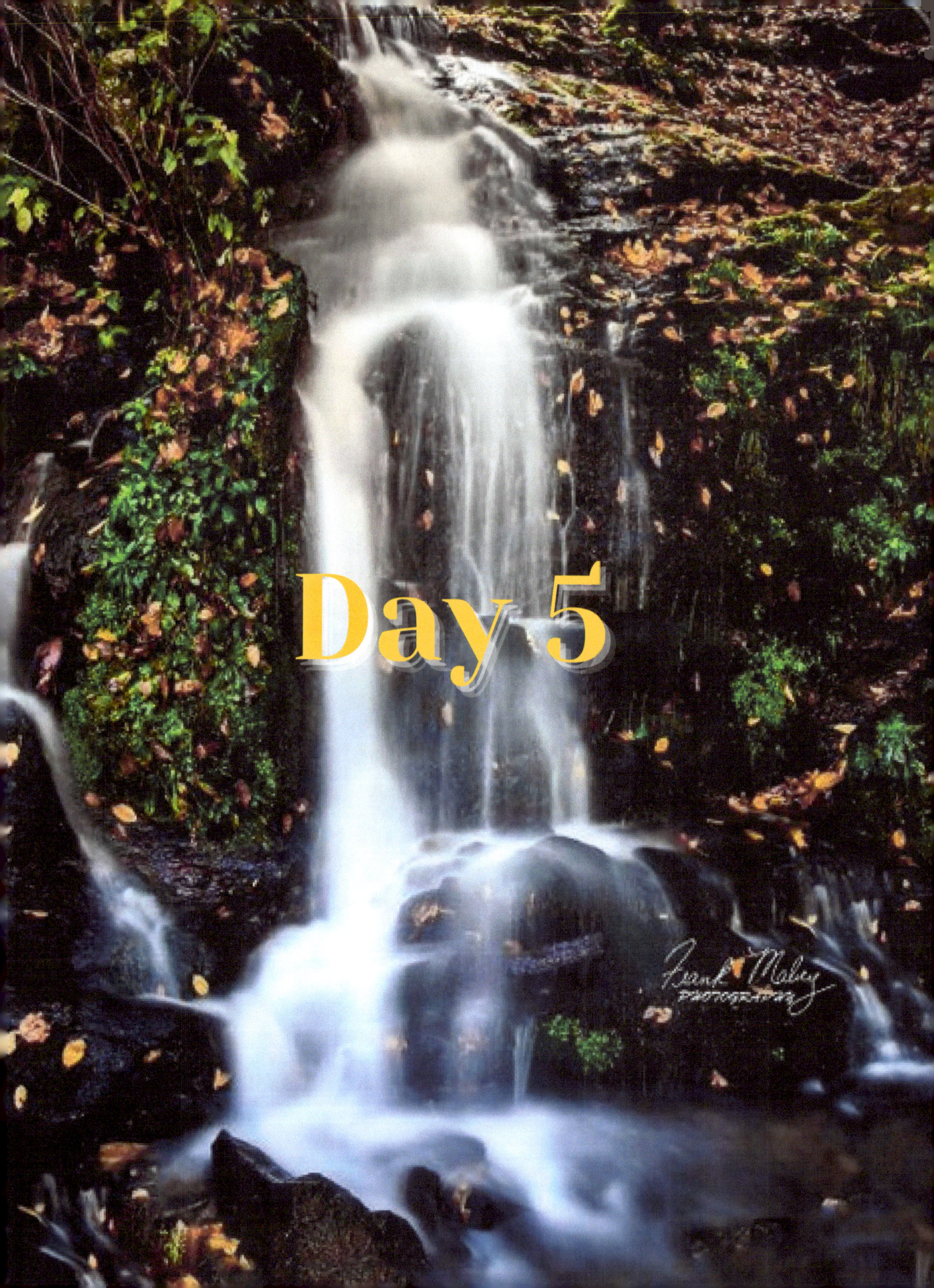

Daily affirmation:

All problems have solutions

Daily scripture:

"The thief's purpose is to steal and kill and destroy. My purpose is to give them a rich and satisfying life."
John 10:10

Daily Petition:

Have mercy upon me and be gracious to me, O Lord; consider how I am afflicted by those who hate me, You who lift me up from the gates of death. Psalm 9:1

Daily act of kindness:
Buy breakfasts for the office

Nutritional recommendation:
Make a fresh smoothie

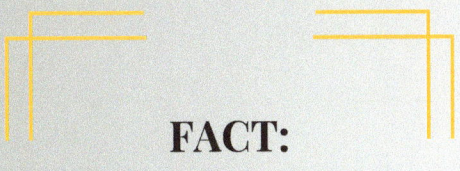

FACT:

Sulfur compounds in onions help to detoxify the body.

Daily Journal

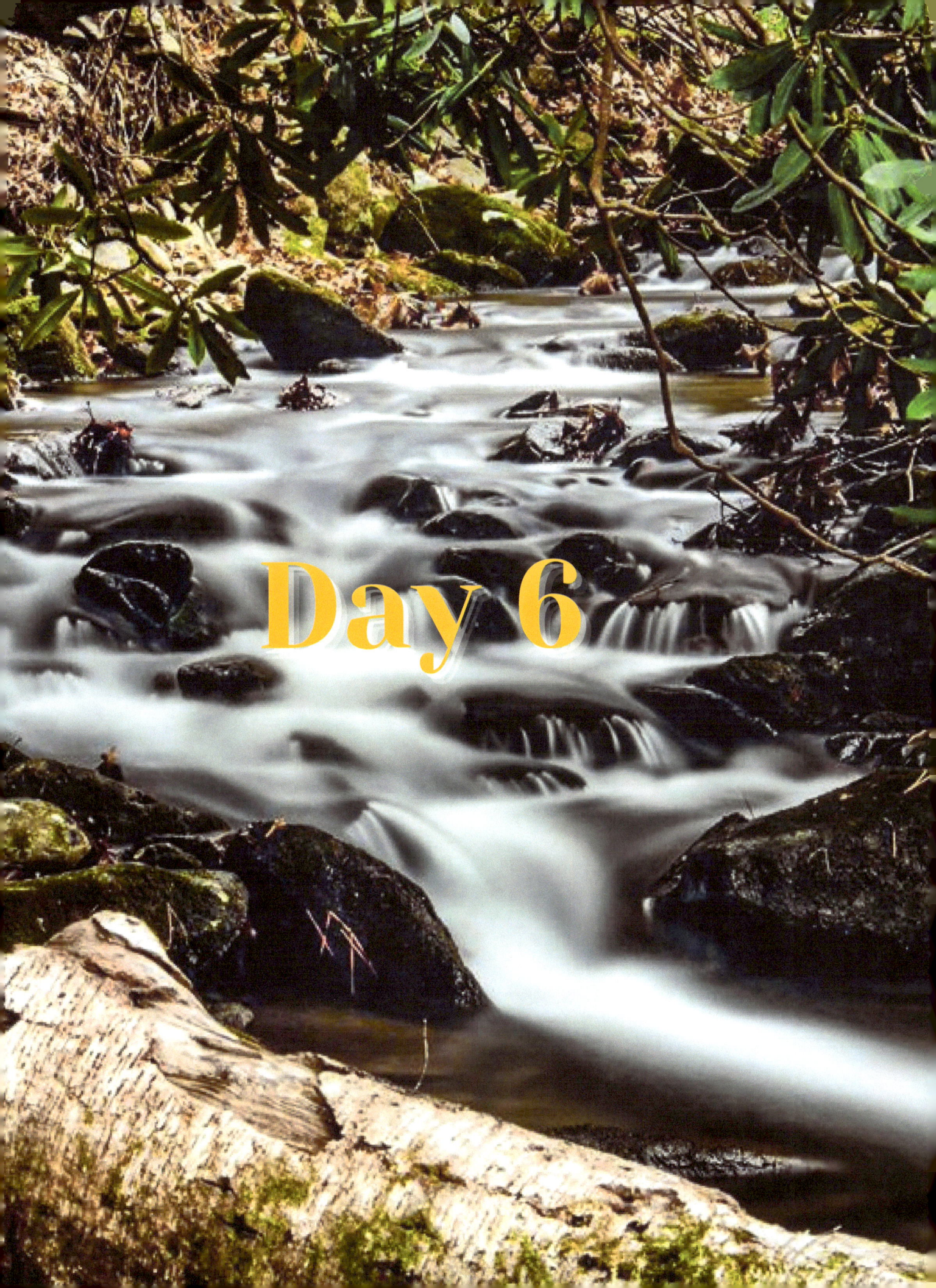

Daily affirmation:

I will treat my body with care and love

Daily scripture:

"A cheerful heart is good medicine, but a crushed spirit dries up bones"
Proverbs 17:22

Daily Petition:

"O Lord My God, in you I take refuge and put my trust; save me from all those who pursue and persecute me, and deliver me."
Psalm 7:1

Daily act of kindness:

Volunteer at your local hospital

Nutritional recommendation:

Try a mediterranean salad

Fact:

Onions are an excellent antioxidant, and they contain anti-allergy, antiviral and antihistamine properties.

Daily Journal

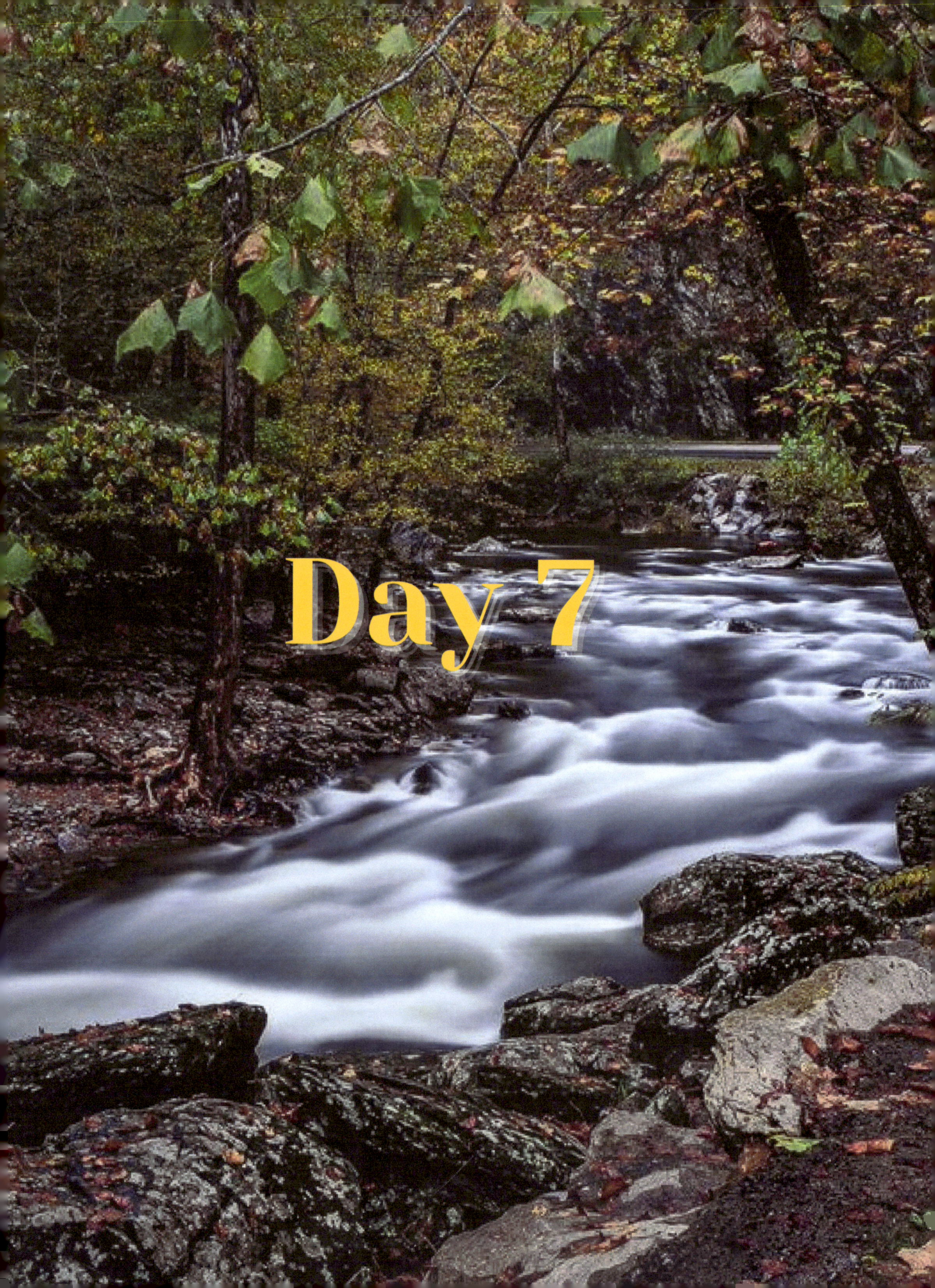

Daily affirmation:

I will let go of negative self-talk

Daily scripture:

"Guard your heart above all else, for it determines the course of your life." Proverbs 4:23

Daily Petition:

Father, give me understanding on dealing with difficult circumstances

Daily act of kindness:

Offer to do something your significant other likes to do

Nutritional recommendation:

Avoid processed meats

Fact:

Green beans are diuretic and may be used to treat diabetes

Daily Journal

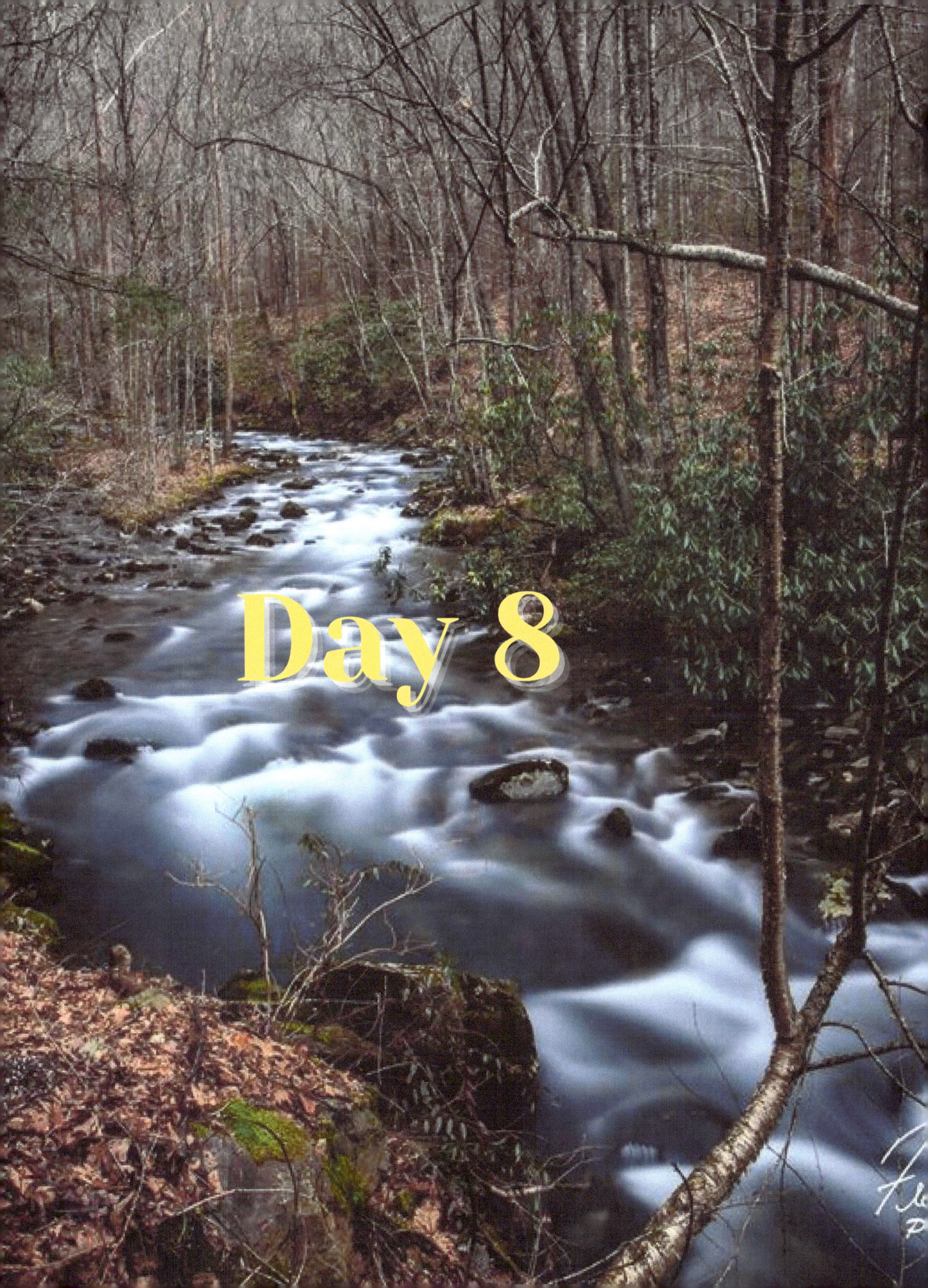

Daily affirmation:

I have the power to create the life I want.

Daily scripture:

"Do not be wise in your own eyes; fear the Lord and shun evil. This will bring health to your body and nourishment to your bones."
Proverbs 3:7-8

Daily Petition:

Heavenly Father remove my fear, doubt and unbelief.

Daily act of kindness:

Volunteer at a nursing home

Nutritional recommendation:

Cook with olive oil

Fact:

Kohlrabi is also high in fiber

Daily Journal

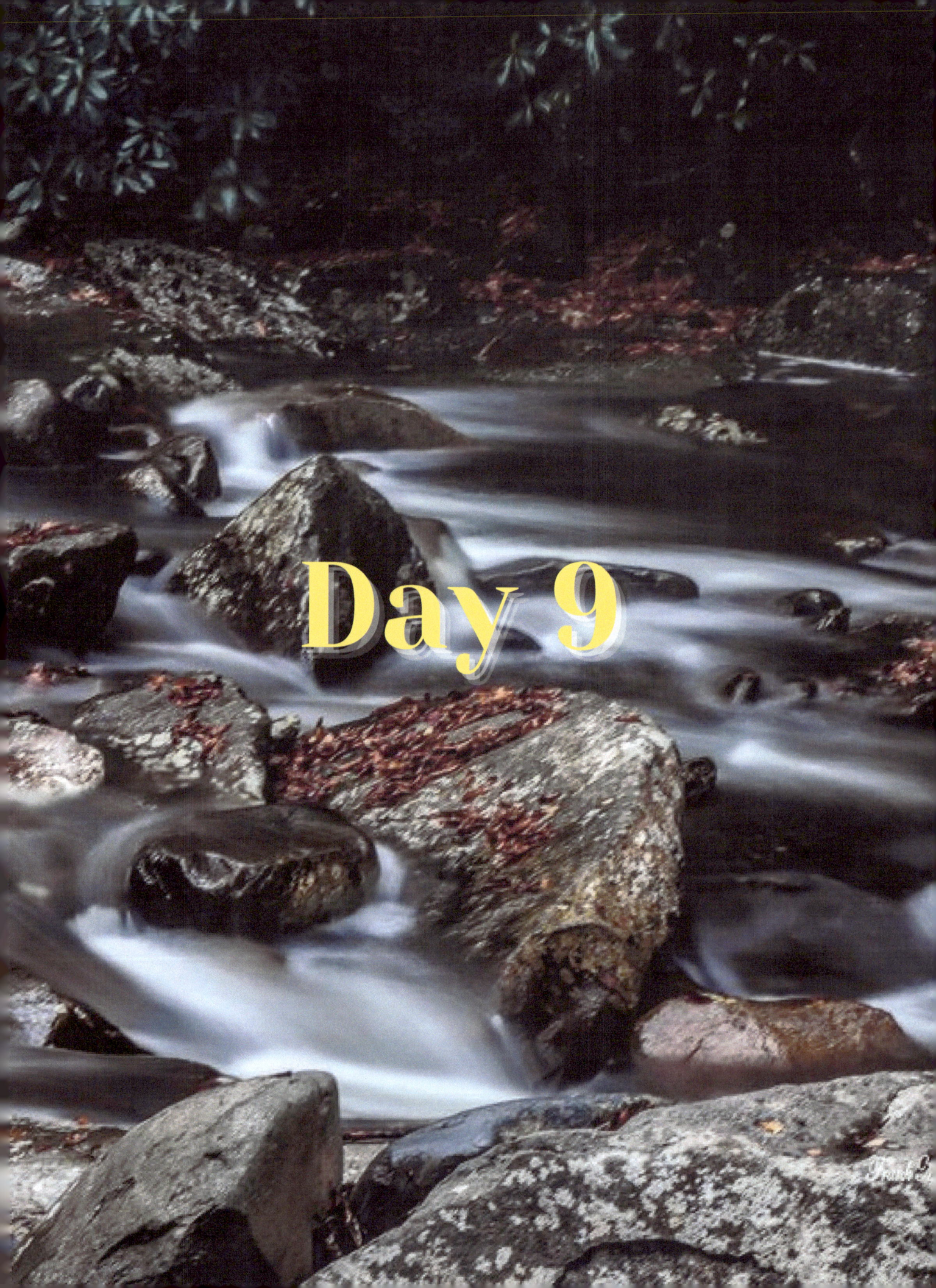

Daily affirmation:

I am supported.

Daily scripture:

"Evening, and morning, and at noon, will I pray, and cry aloud: And he shall hear my voice." Psalm 55:17

Daily Petition:

Father, give me wisdom and understanding.

Daily act of kindness:

Donate school supplies

Nutritional recommendation:

Eliminate as much sugar as possible

Fact:

Mustard may be beneficial for colds, arthritis or depression

Daily Journal

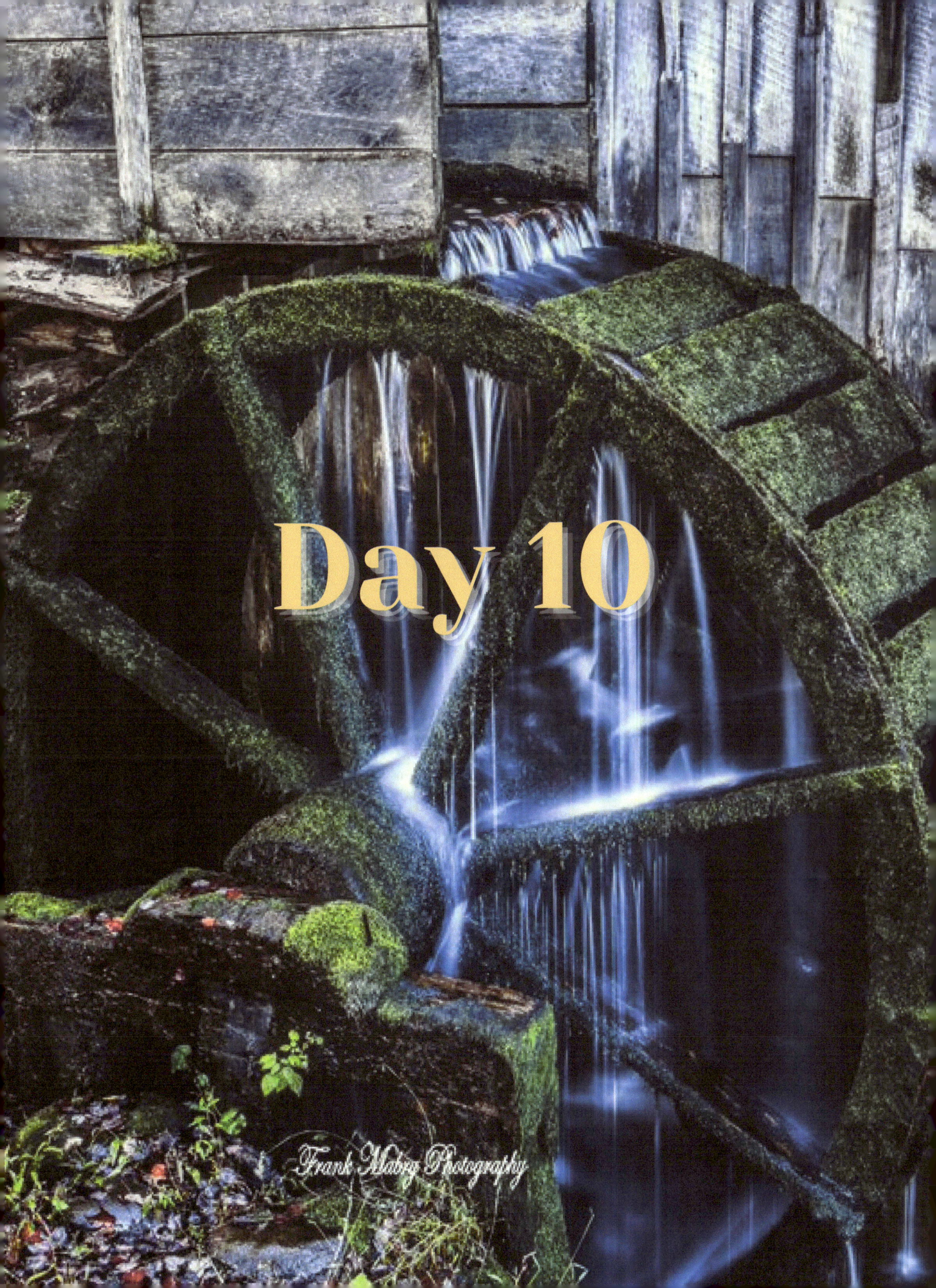

Daily affirmation:

I am strong and I am intlligent

Daily scripture:

"For I know the thoughts that I think towards you, says the Lord, thoughts of peace and not of evil, to give you a future and a hope."
Jeremiah 29:12

Daily Petition:

Father, grant me contentment on this day

Daily act of kindness:

Volunteer at a homeless shelter

Nutritional recommendation:
Eat less saturated fat

Fact:

Potassium is an essential mineral for health. Getting between 3,500 milligrams and 4,700 milligrams a day from tomatoes, spinach, sweet potatoes, and other fruits and vegetables may lower your risk of kidney stones, stroke, and high blood pressure.

Daily Journal

Day 11

frank mabry photography

Daily affirmation:

Every passing day my body is becoming more energetic, more healthy.

Daily scripture:

"Nevertheless, I will bring health and healing to it; I will heal my people and will let them enjoy abundant peace and security." Jeremiah 33:6

Daily Petition:

Father grant me the courage to change the things I no longer can accept.

Daily act of kindness:

Thank a civil servant

Nutritional recommendation:

Replace white rice with quinoa

Fact:

Red dye 40 has been linked to physical and mental health issues.

Daily Journal

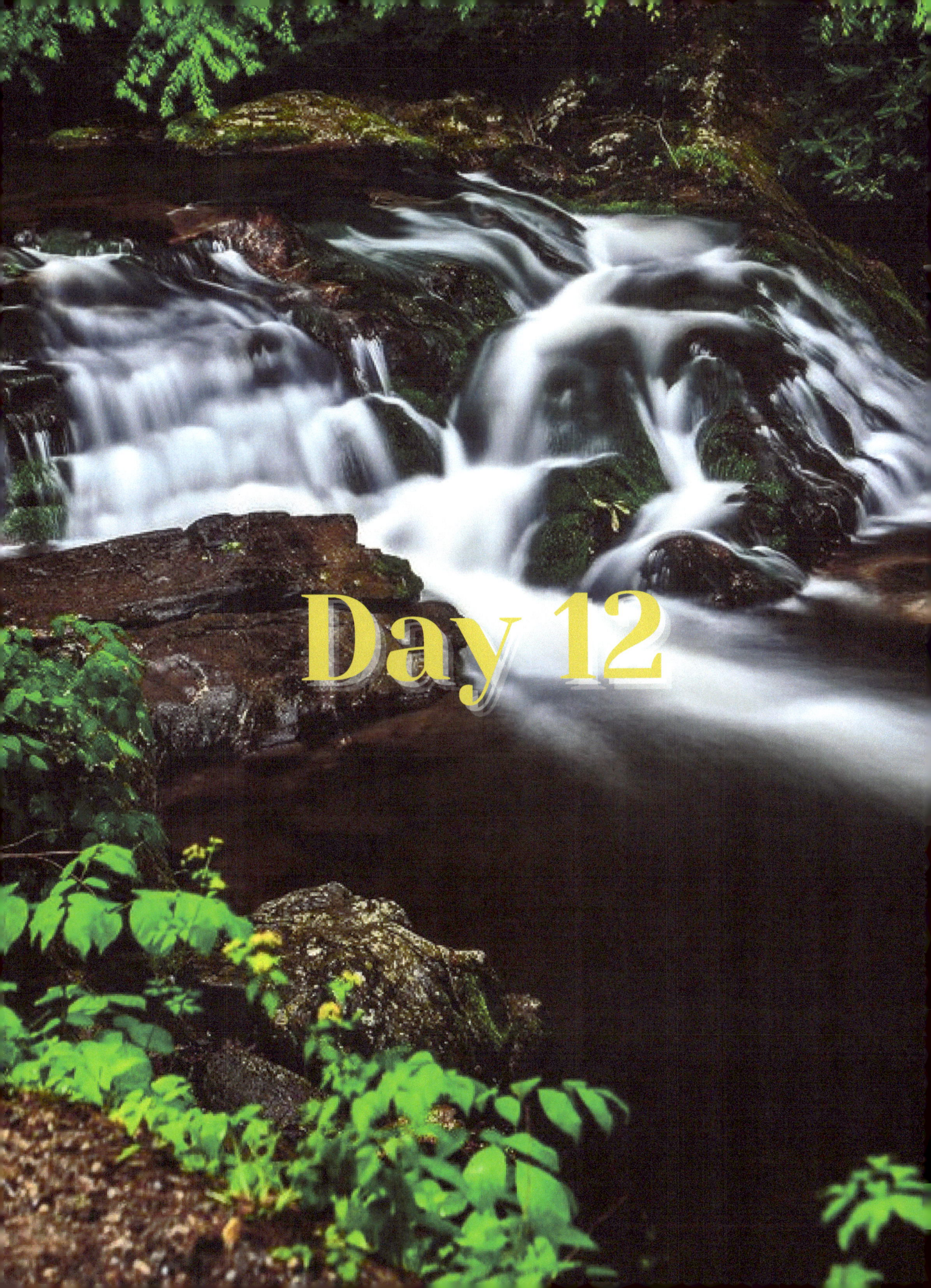

Daily affirmation:

I welcome a sense of calm into my life.

Daily scripture:

"The Lord has heard my plea, the Lord will answer my prayer."
Psalm 6:9

Daily Petition:

Father, order my steps. Show me the path I should walk.

Daily act of kindness:

Help your neighbor with yard work

Nutritional recommendation:

Try sautéed beets as a snack

Fact:

Sucralose may lead to a leaky gut lining, and increase the activity of genes related to inflammation and cancer.

Daily Journal

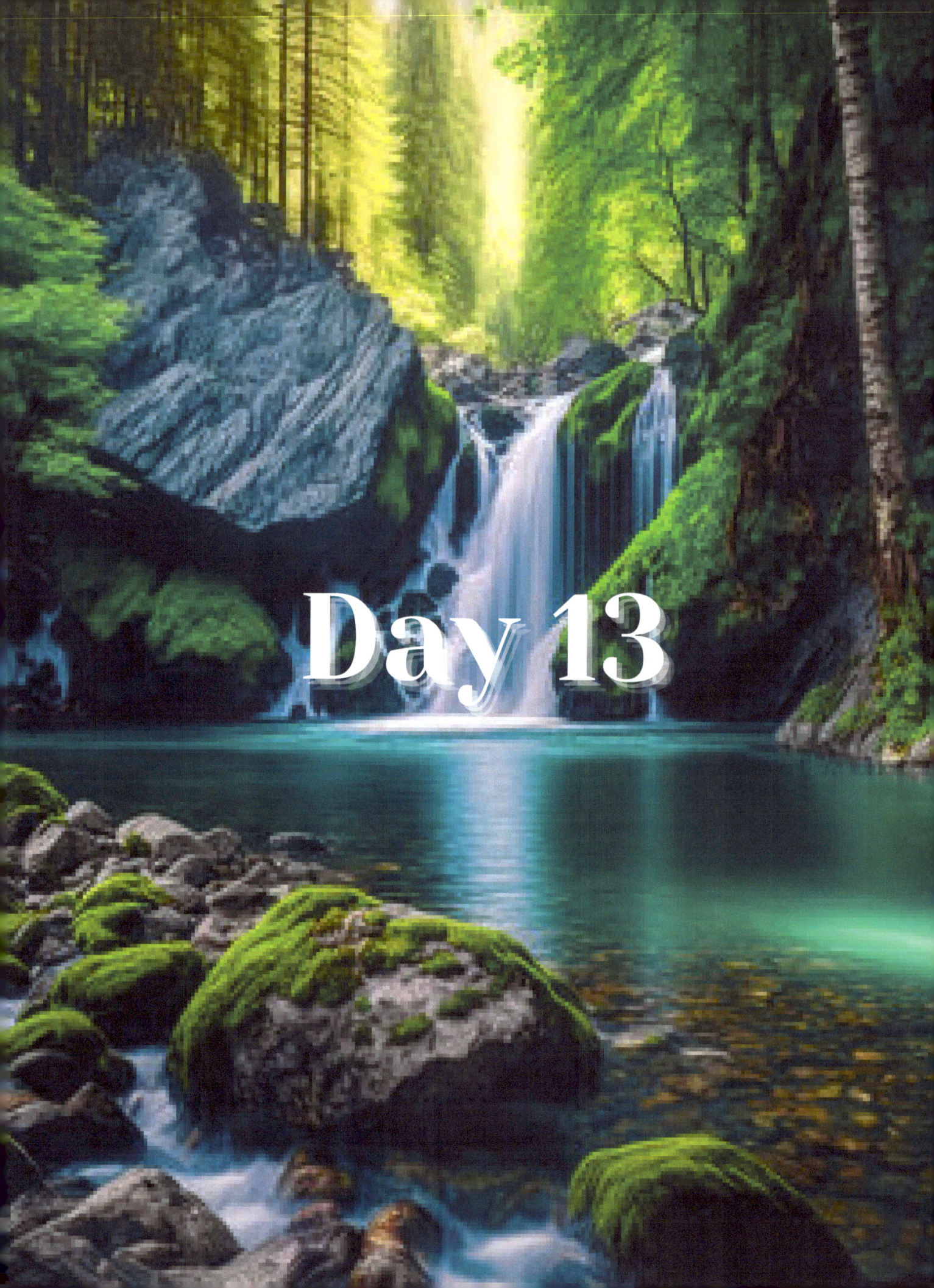

Daily affirmation:

I know my value and will not lessen or shrink myself for anything or anyone.

Daily scripture:

"Pleasant words are as a honeycomb, sweet to the soul, and health to the bones". Proverbs 16:24

Daily Petition:

Father, help me not be anxious about anything.

Daily act of kindness:

Leave a thank-you note for your letter carrier.

Nutritional recommendation:

Try sauteed dinosauer kale with onions

Fact:

Depression alone costs the nation about $210.5 billion annually

Daily Journal

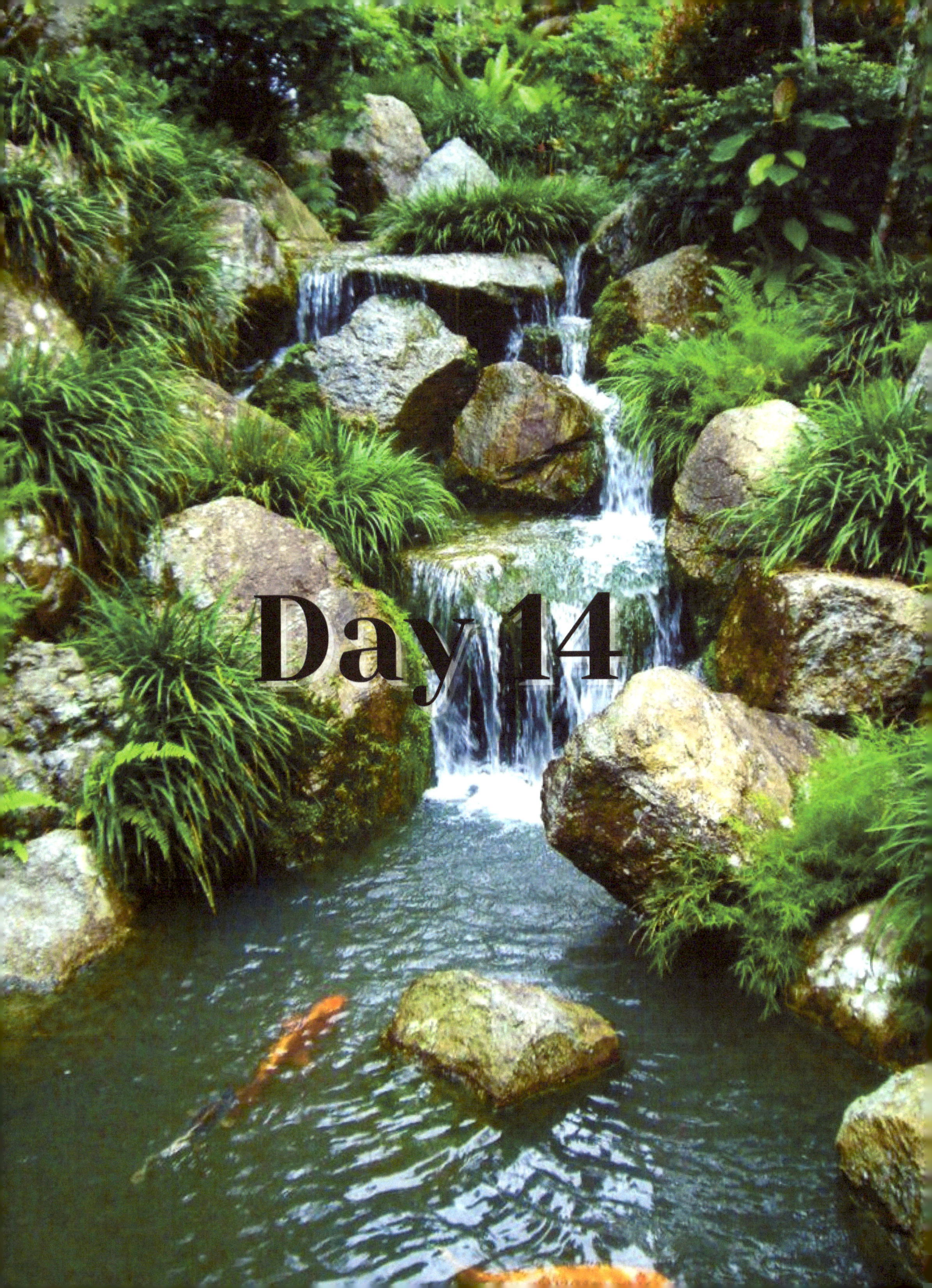

Daily affirmation:

Today I will focus on what makes me feel good.

Daily scripture:

"For my thoughts are not your thoughts, nor are your ways my ways."
Isaiah 55:8

Daily Petition:

Heavenly Father remove my fear, doubt, and unbelief.

Daily act of kindness:

Show compassion to someone who needs it.

Nutritional recommendation:

Try roasted eggplant with Parmesan cheese

Fact:
1 in 5 young people (age 13-18) has or will develop a mental illness in their lifetime.

Daily Journal

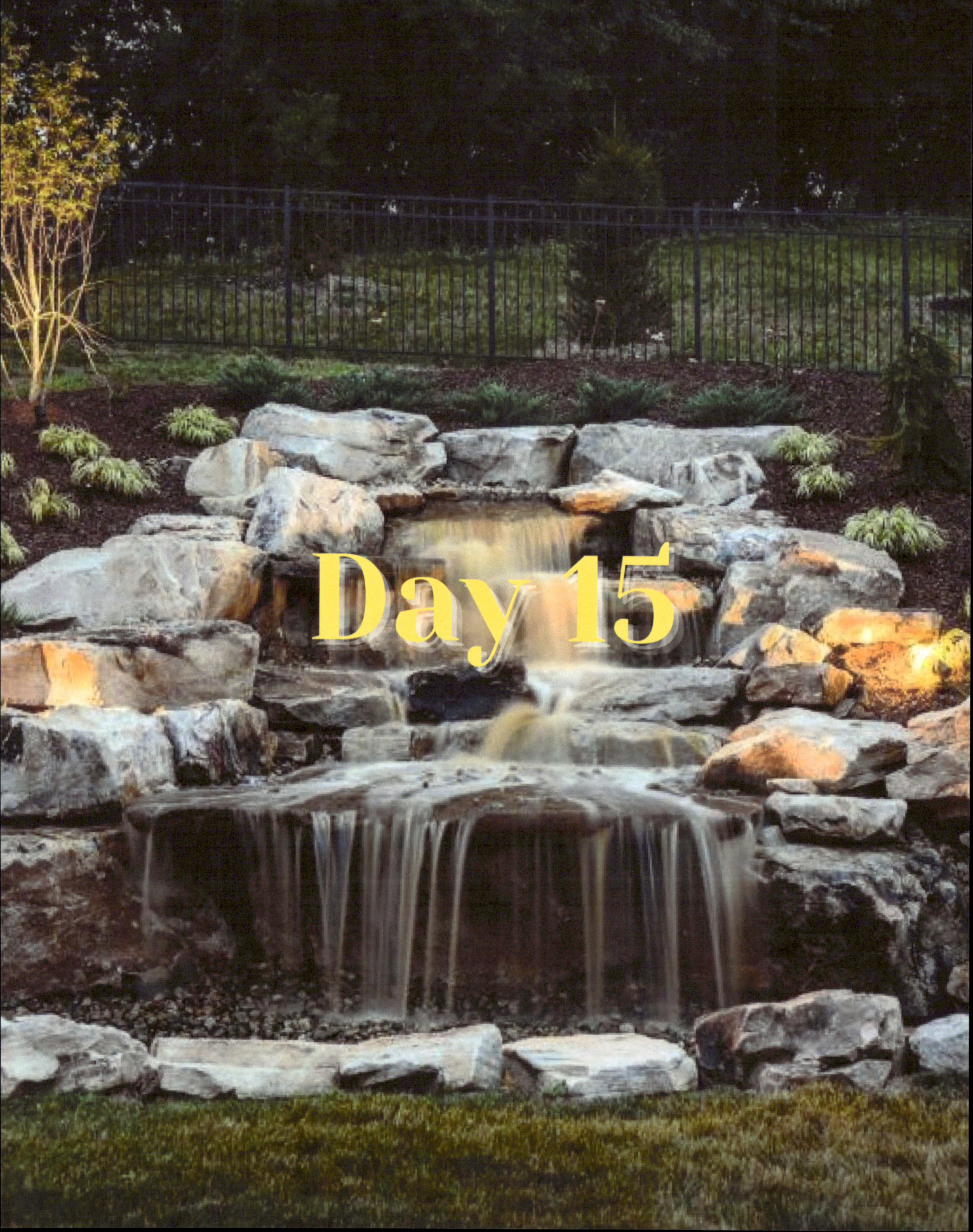

Daily affirmation:

I give myself permission to feel this way without judgment.

Daily scripture:

Cast your anxieties onto the Lord, and He will sustain you.
Psalm 55:22

Daily Petition:

Heavenly Father, help me trust you with my finances.

Daily act of kindness:

Pay for the next person's transaction in line.

Nutritional recommendation:

Limit your consumption of fried foods

Fact:

Maltodextrin, an additive,
widely used in food processing
can raise blood sugar levels

Daily Journal

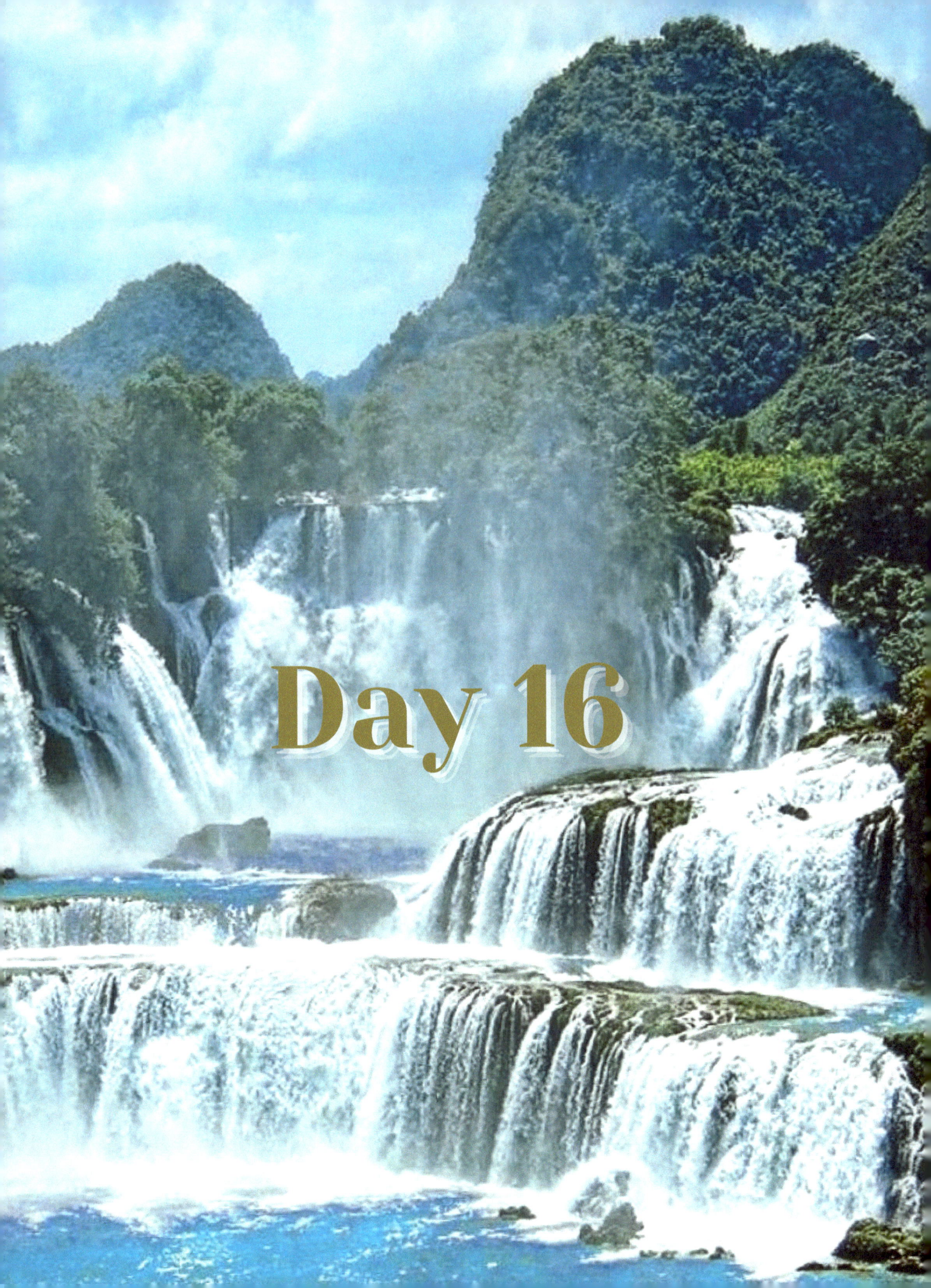

Daily affirmation:

I know my value and will not lessen or shrink myself for anything or anyone..

Daily Scripture:

"I called upon the Lord in distress: The Lord answered me, and set me in a large place." Psalm 118:5

Daily Petition:

Father, allow me to express more gratitude today

Daily act of kindness:

Write a letter/email/text to a family member or friend that you have not reached out to in awhile.

Nutritional recommendation:

Try to eat a vegetable plate today

Fact:

Maternal exposure to high levels of the herbicide glyphosate may increase the risk for autism spectrum disorder (ASD) in offspring; however, the underlying mechanisms remain largely unknown

Daily Journal

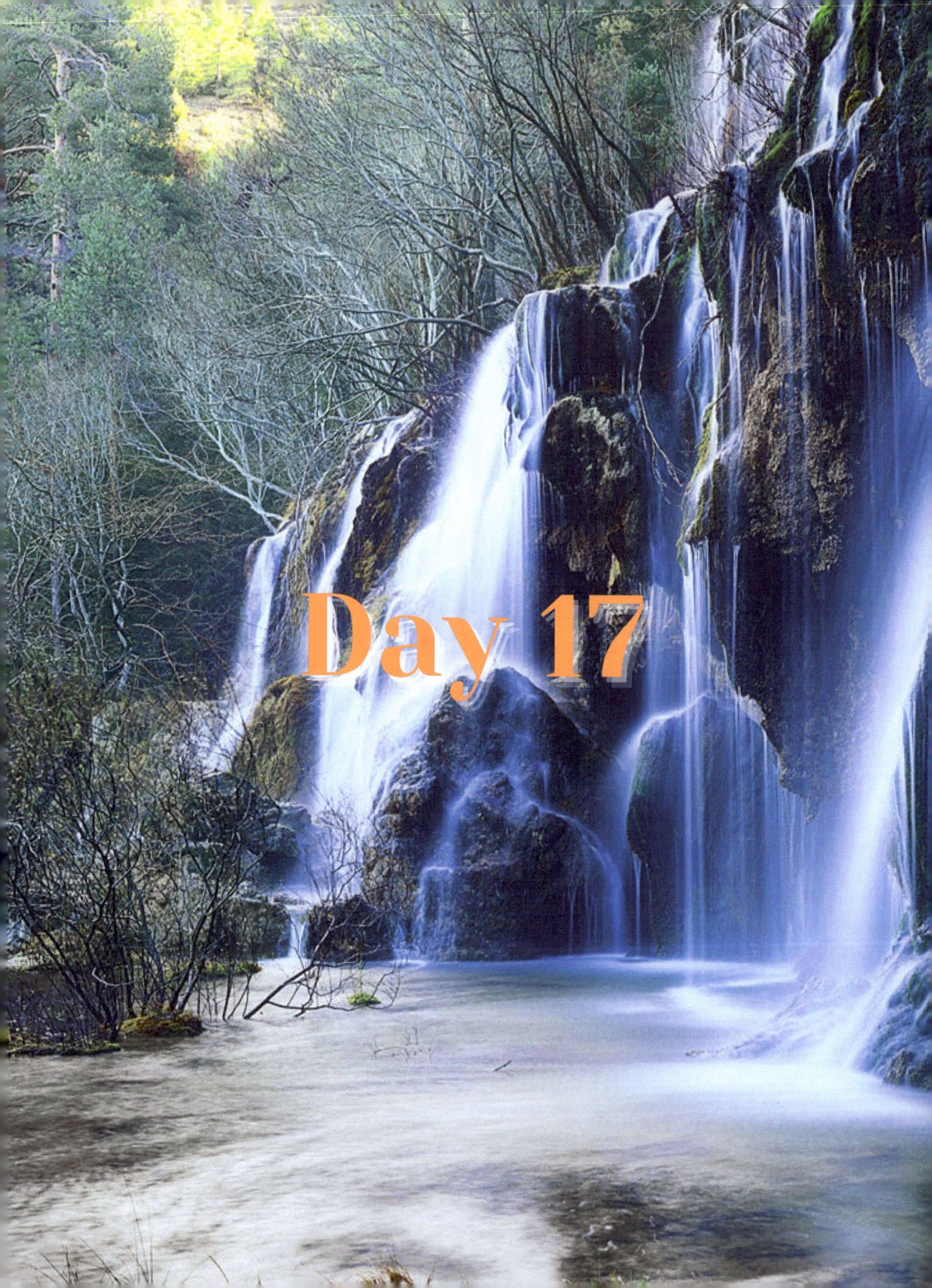

Daily affirmation:

Today I choose to be the very best I can be.

Daily Scripture:

"In whom we have redemption through His blood, the forgiveness of sins." Colossians 1:14

Daily Petition:

Father, I boldly seek you to obtain mercy and to find grace for today

Daily act of kindness:

Pray with a family member, friend or coworker.

Nutritional recommendation:

Try pumpkin seeds for a daily snack

Fact:

Preventive care and annual checkups are necessary for optimal health

Daily Journal

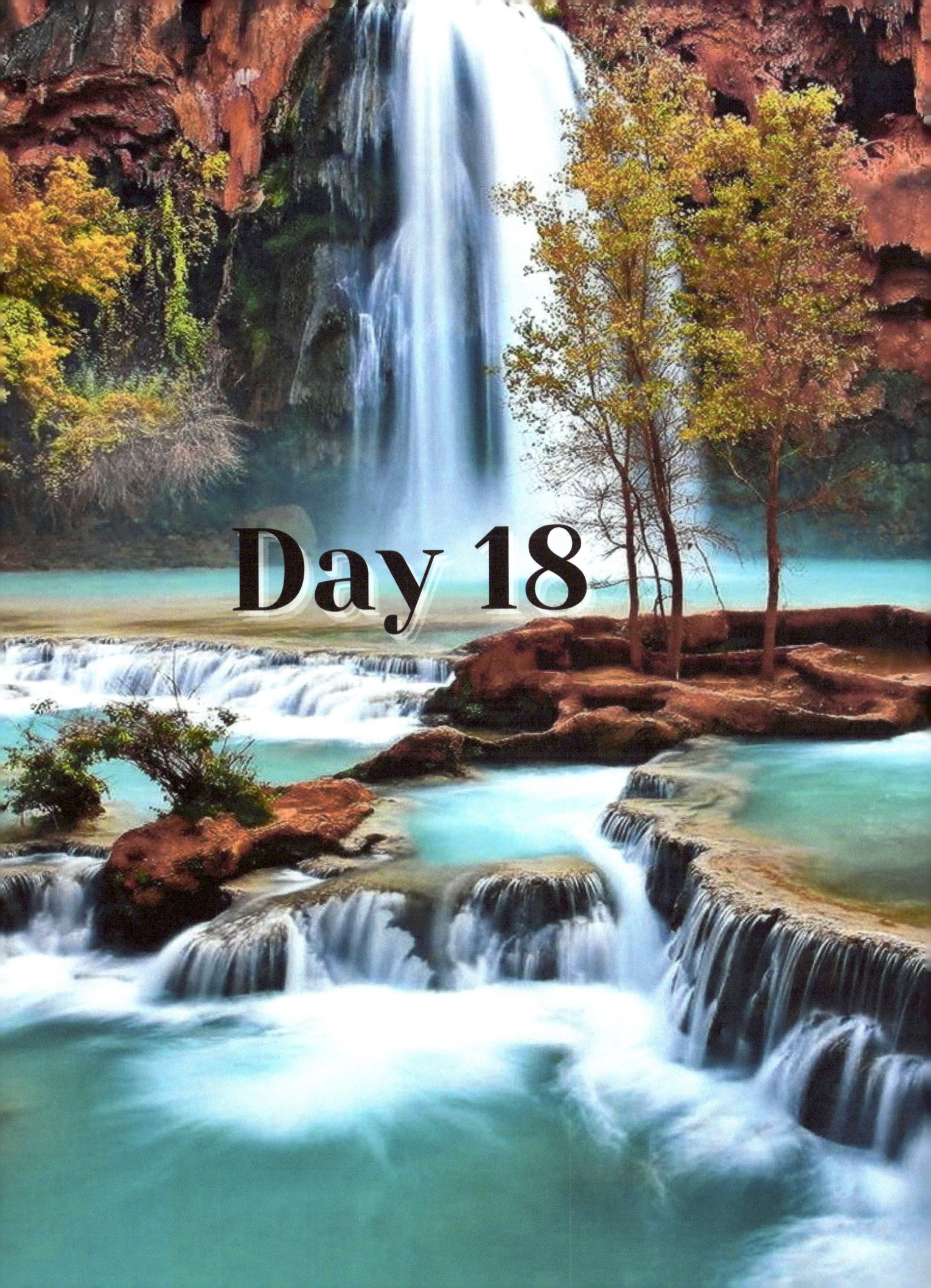

Daily affirmation:
I will renew my mind and think successful thoughts

Daily scripture:
"Two are better than one, because they have a good reward for their labor." Ecclesiastes 4:9

Daily Petition:
Father, grant me wisdom to be the best I can be today.

Daily act of kindness:
Send flowers to a friend..

Nutritional recommendation:
Incorporate a probiotic into your meal plan

Fact:
Females are diagnosed with serious mental health conditions at higher rates males, 7% to 4.2%, respectively

Daily Journal

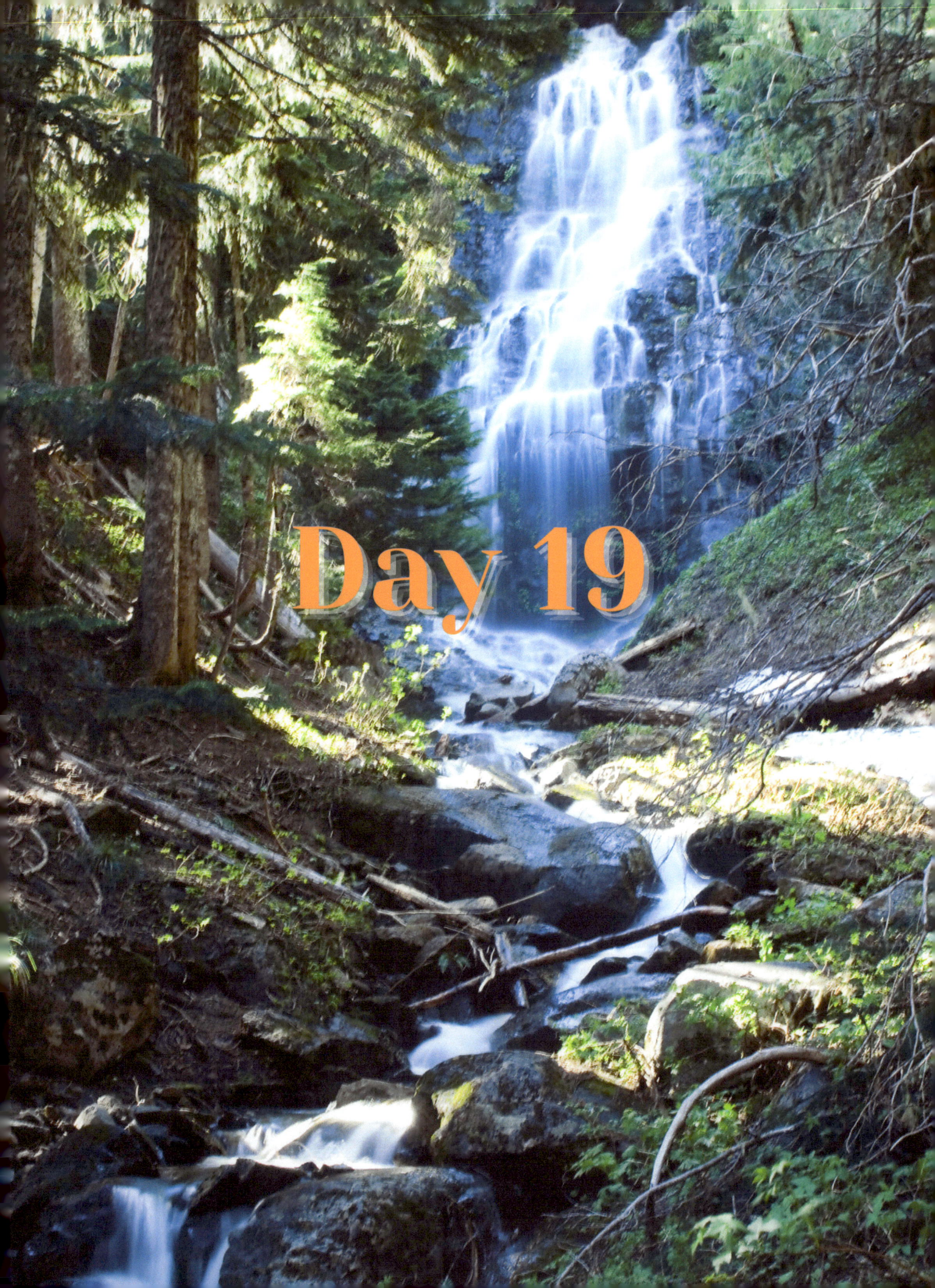
Day 19

Daily affirmation:

I am loved and appreciated even when it seems like I'm not.

Daily scripture:

"Be pleased, O Lord, to deliver me; O Lord, make haste to help me.".
Psalm 40:13

Daily Petition:

Father, give me strength to get through my day.

Daily act of kindness:

Donate financially (and anonymously) to someone in need.

Nutritional recommendation:

Drink a glass of lemon water with breakfast

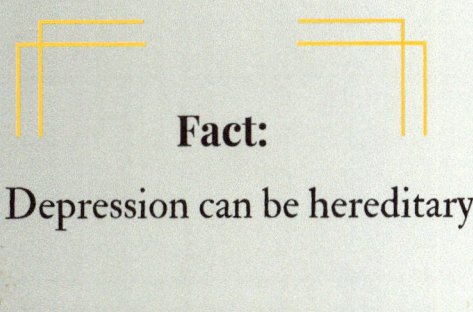

Fact:

Depression can be hereditary

Daily Journal

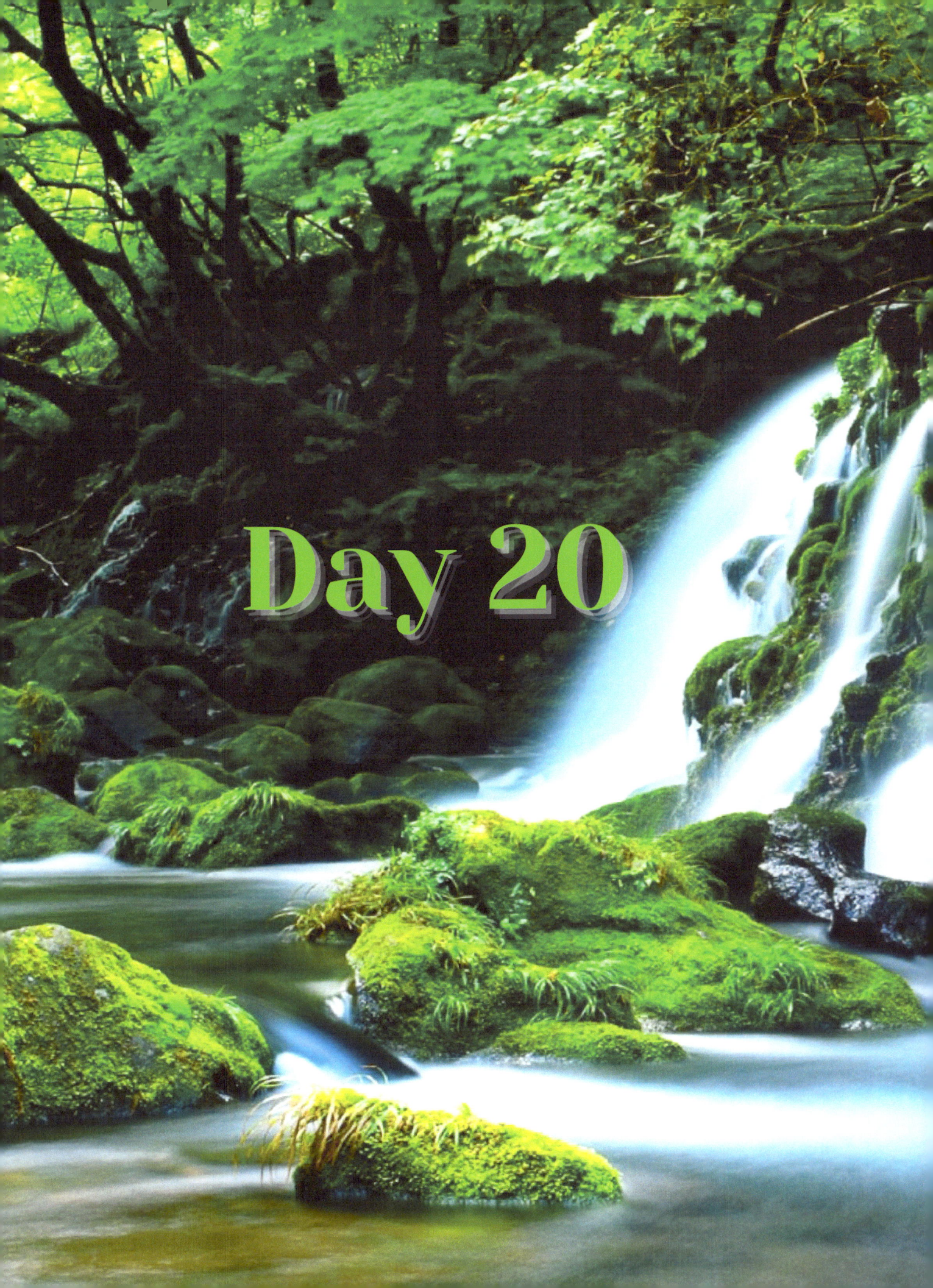

Daily affirmation:

Today, I will remain positive

Daily scripture:

"May mercy, peace, and love be multiplied unto you.".
Jude 1:2

Daily petition:

Father, please remove any hurt, harm, or danger from my path

Daily act of kindness:

Volunteer coaching after school

Nutritional recommendation:

Try making a home-made salad dressing

Fact:

Multiple studies have found a correlation between a diet high in refined sugars and impaired brain function — and even a worsening of symptoms of mood disorders, such as depression.

Daily Journal

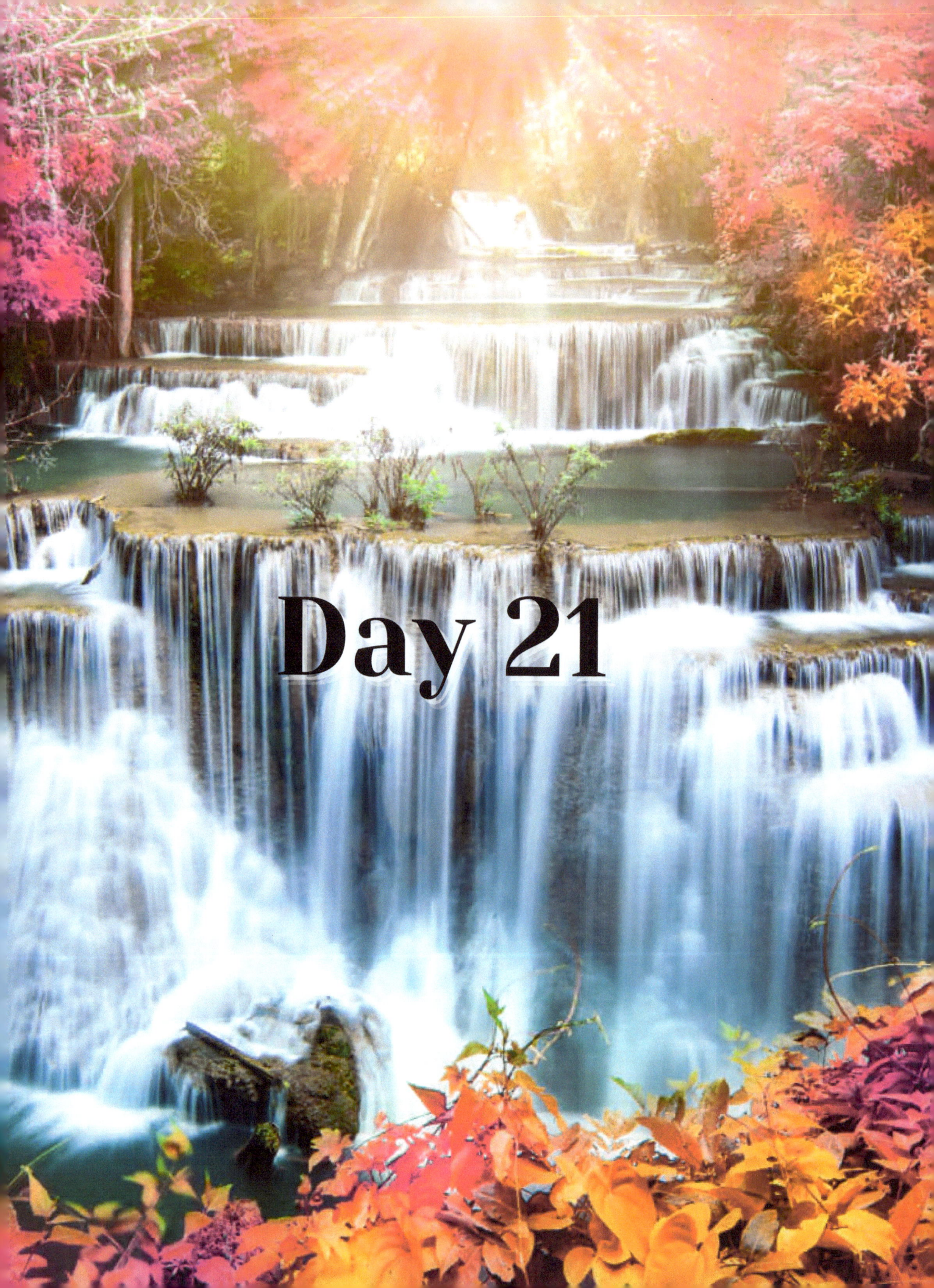

Daily affirmation:

Letting go of worry is becoming easy.

Daily scriptures:

"I waited patiently and expectantly for the Lord, and He inclined to me and heard my cry." Psalm 40:1

Daily petition:

Father, allow me to experience your love today

Daily act of kindness:

Mentor someone for the day.

Nutritional recommendation:

Consider adding a multi-vitamin to your daily routine

Fact:
People who reported their racial identity as two or more races had the highest prevalence of major depressive episodes, at 15.9%

Daily Journal

Recipes

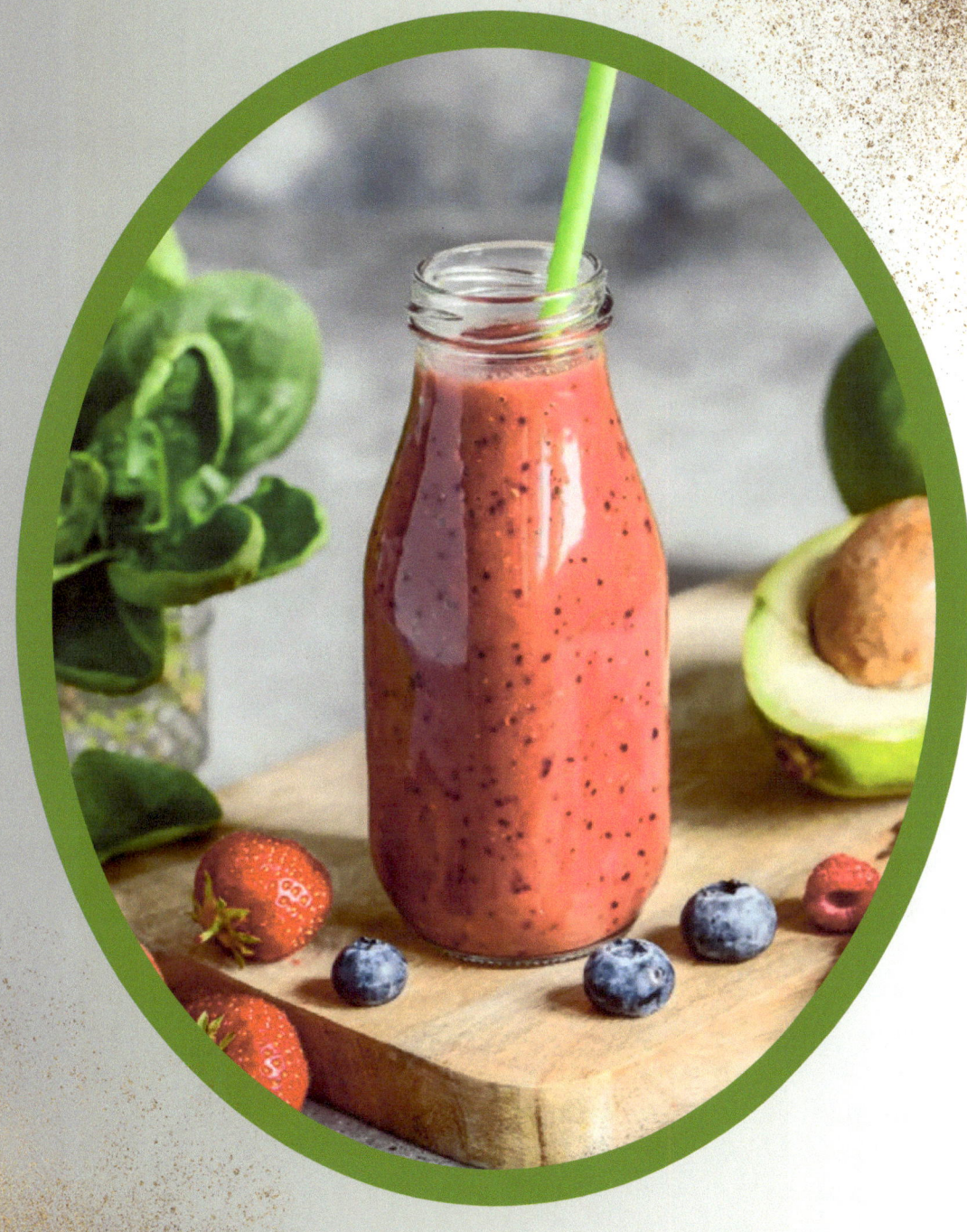

Recipes:

Power Salad

3 cups Arugula/ Bok-Choy

2 cups Spinach

1 cup fresh blueberries

Lemon/ginger salad dressing

1 Tuna pack

1/3 cup fresh onions (optional)

Watermelon (optional)

Mediterranean Power Salad

3 larges leaves of kale

2 cups mixed greens (or other greens of your choice)

1 cup cooked quinoa

1/2 bell pepper, sliced

1/2 cucumber, sliced (optional)

1 whole avocado, sliced

1-2 slices red onion, chopped

1/2 cup marinated artichoke hearts, chopped

10 Kalamata, Picholine, or Green olives

1/3 cup sun-dried tomatoes

Recipes:

Smoothie
(Morning Refresher)

1- organic lemon sliced
1 tsp ginger sliced
1 cup coconut water/ pulp (chilled)
½ tsp of cayenne pepper
1 cup frozen blueberries or pineapple
1 apple organic

Smoothie
(Invigorating)

1-cup of blueberries frozen/fresh
1- Tbsp ginger grated
1- cup pomegranate juice
½ cup Dinosaur kale chopped
1 tsp honey
1/2 cup ice
Pumpkin seeds for a snack

Recipes:

Smoothie
(Power-up)

1 scoop Protein Powder
1 small banana/ organic
½ cup blueberries frozen
½ cup peanut butter / organic
1 cup coconut/pineapple water(chilled)
1 cup greek vanilla yogurt

Smoothie
(Mindfulness)

½ cup kale
½ cup spinach
2 oz dark chocolate
½ cup of frozen strawberries
1 cup of blueberries frozen
8-12 oz sparkling water
1 tbsp chia seeds
1 to 2 oz of walnuts for a snack

Please provide feedback on your 21-Day journal by scanning the QR-Code below with phone camera or scan option in your settings.

Thank you for completing the Mental Health and Wellness Journal. We look forward to providing you with more products and service.

KMM is eternally grateful to those that helped make this book happen. A special thank you to:
Digital Creators- Ethan Brown & Bryce Bryant
Photographer- Frank Mabry